Diabetes Care
for Babies, Toddlers,
and Preschoolers
A Reassuring Guide

About the Author

Jean Betschart, MSN, CRNP, CPNP, CDE, is a pediatric nurse practitioner and diabetes educator in the Department of Endocrinology, Diabetes and Metabolism at Children's Hospital of Pittsburgh. She is also a member of the adjunct faculty at the University of Pittsburgh Department of Health Promotion and Development. She has worked with children with diabetes and their families since 1980, and has had Type 1 diabetes for over 30 years. She is also a past president of the American Association of Diabetes Educators and was named Educator of the Year in 1994 by the American Diabetes Association. Ms. Betschart has written numerous books, chapters, and articles on diabetes for children, parents, and health care professionals.

Also by Jean Betschart

It's Time to Learn about Diabetes, ages 8–11
John Wiley & Sons

A Magic Ride in Foozbah-Land, ages 3–7
John Wiley & Sons

In Control: a Guide for Teens with Diabetes, ages 14 and up
John Wiley & Sons

Raising a Child with Diabetes (ADA)
50 Ways to Manage Diabetes (International Publications)

Diabetes Care
for Babies, Toddlers,
and Preschoolers
A Reassuring Guide

Jean Betschart, CRNP, CDE

JOHN WILEY & SONS, INC.

New York • Chichester • Weinheim • Brisbane • Singapore • Toronto

This book is printed on acid-free paper. ☉

Copyright © 1999 by Jean Betschart. All rights reserved
Published by John Wiley & Sons, Inc.
Published simultaneously in Canada
Previously published by Chronimed Publishing

Illustrations: Pat Rouse

The information contained in this book is not intended to serve as a
replacement for professional medical advice. Any use of the information in this
book is at the reader's discretion. The author and the publisher specifically
disclaim any and all liability arising directly or indirectly from the use or
application of any information contained in this book. A health care
professional should be consulted regarding your specific situation.

Library of Congress Cataloging-in-Publication Data:

ISBN 0-471-34676-4

Printed in the United States of America

10   9   8   7   6   5   4   3   2

Contents

Acknowledgments

With deepest affection, I acknowledge the support and love of my family and friends who have encouraged this effort. Special thanks goes to my husband, Jim, for his never ending patience and willingness to help in any capacity.

As a parent, there can be little in this world that we love more than our children. Therefore, I dedicate this book to my own children and to all parents of children with diabetes.

I gratefully appreciate the following contributors and reviewers for their interest, support, and wonderful suggestions: Catherine Bellis; Marilyn Clougherty, MSN, CDE; Beth Ann Coonrod, PhD, RN, CDE; David Finegold, MD; Sally Foster, MSN, CDE; Stacy and Tony Karabinos; Karen Kelly, BSN, CDE; Terri Travis, MS, RD, CDE; and Ellen Warner.

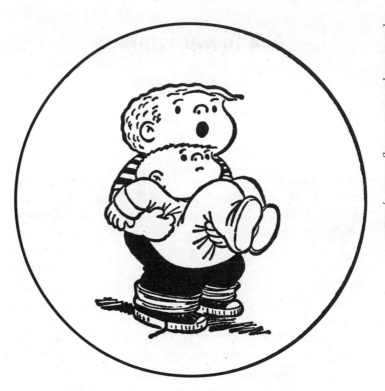

Mommy, how long did it take me to grow up?

Introduction

PARENTS OF LITTLE ONES with newly diagnosed diabetes describe taking their child home from the hospital as much worse than taking a new baby home from the hospital. There are instructions, diabetes paraphernalia, things to do, things to organize, and things to read, in addition to all of the normal parenting stuff. The health care team, your family, and your friends all may have expectations. Your own expectations are often greater than everyone else's. Anxiety about learning it all or about doing something that could harm your child are common feelings.

If your child is in day care or preschool, the staff also has many of these same concerns. If you don't feed a newborn on time or miss a messy diaper for a while, well, although not desirable, it happens. But if you don't feed a baby with diabetes on time, or don't recognize hypoglycemic signs, there could be trouble. In spite of this, however, be reassured that there is not much that you could do to cause great harm as long as you are taking reasonable care and making sound judgments based on your knowledge. There is little that can happen that cannot be rather quickly corrected, and most of the time our understanding of what would have worked better comes as hindsight. As you become familiar and comfortable with the diabetes routine and your child's response to it, the whole family can relax with confidence in knowledge, understanding, and an optimistic outlook.

Understanding normal development and the effect diabetes has on it is important in managing a young child with diabetes. In general, children younger than six years old are different from school-age children in a lot of ways. Each stage brings physical, mental, and emotional changes. Foods and eating patterns change as babies are weaned from breast or bottle and begin to eat solid foods. Blood glucoses vary according to sporadic eating and activity.

You were probably told that your child should have insulin within a certain time period and eat the same amount of food at regular times. You were most likely told to test your child's blood glucose regularly, to know when it is important to call your doctor, to write it all down, and to be able to observe for and treat signs of low blood glucose. These tasks usually sound overwhelming at first, but are quite "do-able," as many parents of little ones will testify. Somehow, they become a way of life. Sometimes it is a matter of organization to get it all pulled together, sometimes it's a matter of energy, and sometimes it's a matter of support. And sometimes, what you do just doesn't go as expected.

As a parent, you will change as you face the issues of diabetes care. At first you may have all of the usual feelings of grief, including sadness. You may also be eager to learn, but then as you slowly realize the reality of the amount of responsibility and care involved you can become frightened. You may shake your head, trying to clear the emotional fog and understand the meaning of it all, determined to take the best care of your child. And yet, you may be full of fear, anxiety, and concern about how to fit it all into your life. There is no question that the tasks that you are about to do are difficult. You will, most likely, not be able to do all of the tasks in the best way, all of the time. You will get quite tired of it at times. However, if you liken the diabetes journey to a race, it is not a sprint; it is a marathon. You will need to pace yourself, be a good steward of your energy and reserves, and learn not to be hard on yourself when things are not going exactly right.

It is very important as a parent or caretaker of a very young child with diabetes that your child has excellent medical care. Because pediatric diabetes is a very specialized area and because young children require greater and different expertise than older children, infants, toddlers, and preschool children should be followed at a multidisciplinary team diabetes center that specializes in pediatric diabetes, or by a pediatric endocrinologist. The team should include a physician, nurse educator, dietitian, and psychologist or social worker. These professionals will be able to give you the information and support you need. If you find that you live far from a major center and do not have transportation, it can often be worked out that you visit them once or twice a year with in-between visits to your primary care doctor, and communicate by phone or fax if it is available to you.

As a parent, diabetes management can be confusing because you may get mixed messages from different health care professionals. Not everyone approaches diabetes in the same way. Different diabetes centers and different diabetes specialists in the same center will often approach diabetes differently. As a parent, you need to integrate these approaches into what works for you and your child, keeping in mind that parents and health care professionals have similar goals. Both are on the same team, striving for a healthy, happy child and family, normal growth and development, and ultimately, a successful school performance. As a parent, however, you are the advocate for your young child. Your health care team is also an advocate for you and your child to the greater community. You will need to find a balance between good diabetes management and normal family life. The word *normal* here may cause you to balk, saying, "Normal, how can all of this ever be normal?" As one dad put it, "There just becomes a new kind of 'normal.'" The goal is to incorporate good diabetes care into your family life in the easiest way possible.

The care of a young child with diabetes, as for all people with diabetes, is individualized. Suzy's diabetes program may appear quite different from Mark's even though they are exactly the same age. Suzy is a good eater, moderately active, likes a schedule, demands a nap, and tolerates injections fairly well. Mark, on the other hand, refuses to eat breakfast, is highly active, never naps, and fights injections with every ounce of his being. If your two-year-old will tolerate injections in legs but howls at arm injections, there are compromises that can be made in the rotation pattern for injections. Adjustments in insulin and food timing will need to be made to adjust the treatment program to each child's characteristics and temperament.

This book is not intended to present everything you need to know about managing diabetes in an infant and toddler. But it will help you understand how diabetes impacts normal development in young children, give you ideas for problemsolving that have worked for other parents, and give you tips that will help fit diabetes demands into real-life schedules. Some things may work; some may not. After reading this book, you should have a better understanding of how diabetes affects your child and have plenty of ideas for dealing with routine diabetes care in your child. Children seem to know when their parents are tense or anxious, which can contribute to the general level of anxiety in the home. The goal is to learn, understand, and develop a structured yet flexible approach so that you and your family can all relax in the security of your knowledge and ability.

Parents who have contributed to this book have done so generously and willingly to try to help others benefit from their wealth of knowledge and practical experience. They want you to know that someday you will look back and wonder how you did it! You will have done it and done it well.

Diabetes Care
for Babies, Toddlers,
and Preschoolers

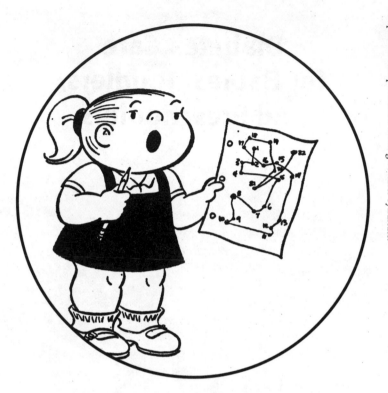

"*I made up a connect-the-dots picture,
but when I connected the dots, nothing came out.*"

CHAPTER I

Getting a Grip

WHEN YOUR CHILD is first diagnosed with diabetes, there is a lot to handle. Thoughts and emotions whirl, family and friends (though often quite helpful) can complicate matters with their thoughts and opinions. You are most likely exhausted. Try to understand that all of this is quite common and that it will take you some time to get back on track and heal.

Dealing with the loss

It is well known that when children become sick or have a chronic illness, their parents usually feel a great sense of loss. When our children are born, or even before birth, we have dreams and expectations of what they will be like. Will they be tall or short? Fat or thin? Blue eyes or brown? Athlete? Professor? Happily married with children? Nowhere in our vision is the thought that they may have diabetes. When diabetes hits, there is naturally some mental adjusting that must happen. Thoughts of what Jenny might be like when she grows up now must include the acknowledgment that she has a chronic illness, and not an easy one at that. Thoughts race to questions such as, "What will her life be like in twenty years?" "How will diabetes affect her personality or appearance?" "Will she be sickly?" "Will she fall in love and get married?" "Will she be able to pursue the career of her choice?" "Will she be able to have healthy babies if she wants?" "What if we don't do a good job at this diabetes control?" "What if she rebels?" "How will her temperament, personality, and academic or athletic performance be affected?" "What about complications?"

These questions are normal and natural. If you can contain the explosion of anxiety that they create, however, it will help you deal with them better.

Ellen Warner, a parent, commented, "We also worried that the happy, silly little child we took to the hospital would be changed when we took him home. Would he also sense the loss? Our answer was that he was still a happy, funny guy. Maybe a child's strange sense of reality means that they make the adjustment more readily than parents."

Of course, no one knows what is down the road for any of us. The best we can do is to take one step at a time, one day at a time. Reassurance will come. Your child, and perhaps life itself, seems quite vulnerable to you. It takes some time to adjust to the notion that Jenny is still your perfect child...and she also has diabetes.

Of course there are additional losses that can happen when a child gets diabetes. Parents may have less time together, less time for leisure activity, and less freedom, and relationships can become strained. If you don't have good health care insurance coverage, money can also become a loss as the treatment for diabetes is costly.

As you realize these losses, it is common for many parents to feel depressed, lonely, or isolated. Feelings like this are normal and are part of the process of dealing with a loss. Usually, with patience, time, and outside support, they fade. Give yourself permission to be sad. It is OK to cry. Try to accept love, hugs and help from others. They want to help and don't know how. In time, you may need to develop some strategies to deal with these feelings, such as planning a "date night" out without children, joining a support group for parents, going to counseling, finding ways to relax and have fun, and relying on spiritual help.

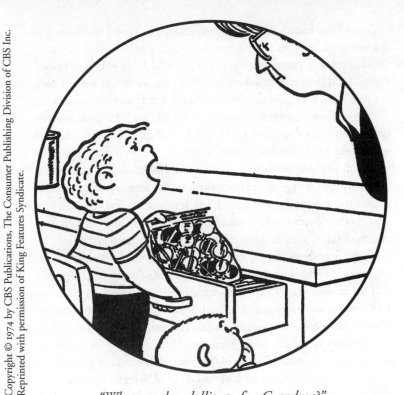

"What are these lollipops for, Grandma?"

Family feuds or family fun?

When an illness like diabetes occurs in a child, it can cause some major changes in family behavior. Of course most family members are concerned and want to help, but sometimes it takes a little skill to straighten out misconceptions and false information, and get everyone going in the same direction. Grandparents, aunts, uncles, dozens of cousins, and close friends can descend on you, each with their own opinion about how things should go. Sometimes there is a lot of blaming that goes on as Aunt Millie remembers that diabetes came from one side of the family or the other, and that your great aunt on your mother's side had diabetes and died at an early age. The bottom line is that no one is to blame for the diabetes. Although the chance of developing diabetes can be predicted fairly accurately with genetic typing, there is little that can be done to prevent it, and it is no one's fault.

If you have friends or relatives with adult, or Type 2, diabetes, you may have to deal with their misunderstanding of diabetes in a young child. To many people, diabetes is diabetes. They may not understand the differences between Type 2 diabetes, where weight control, exercise, pills, and sometimes insulin are treatment, and Type 1 diabetes, where insulin therapy is a must. Frequently, there are misunderstandings about what should and shouldn't be eaten, how often, and when. And of course, when the person with Type 1 is a young child there are a whole set of developmental issues that sometimes are not recognized. It is common for those with experience with Type 2 diabetes to want to restrict calories and fat, and provide dietetic foods in the meal plan, which is not appropriate for a young child. Children need enough calories to keep growing.

Other friends and family members who can pose difficulty are the well-meaning but less-than-helpful relatives who come to help but end up in your way. These folks may hover, take up your time, actually create work for you, or sometimes even sabotage your diabetes efforts. They come out of good will, interest, or concern, but may not be eager or able to learn what must be done to take care of diabetes. Or, they may provide inappropriate foods at inappropriate times for your child because your child shouldn't feel deprived. This is the person who announces that "just one little piece won't hurt!" (Sweets are listed at the top of the food pyramid and everyone should follow the "use sparingly" tip.)

Even though they are well intentioned, you will need to learn to protect yourself from intrusiveness and anything else that leads to poor diabetes care. The first priority is the health and well-being of your family. You will need to be strong and consistent to deal with them in the best possible way.

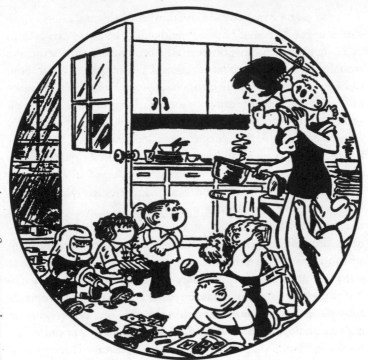

*"Melanie and Buddy came over here to play
'cause their mommy is readin' a book."*

Taking action

One of the best ways to help your family and friends help you is to tell them exactly what you need. Sometimes this can be difficult if you are not in the habit of asking for help. One mother said that when Aunt Sally offered help, "I just asked her if she could take Jenny and Jessie out on Thursday afternoon while I took Sam to the doctor. She seemed happy to help. Otherwise she might have shown up on the doorstep with a chocolate cake, which none of us need." You might want to ask a relative to:

- bring you a pot of soup, or pick up milk from the store;
- learn how to do finger pricks, give injections, and treat hypoglycemia;
- take your kids to scouts;
- baby-sit so that you can go to a movie or take a nap.

Try to become assertive about asking for help, and build a delegation of good helpers. Finding good child care these days is difficult enough, but finding someone who is trained to understand and treat diabetes can be even more difficult. Learning all you can about diabetes and its care will help you have a good foundation to teach others. You may do some of your own teaching, or there may be diabetes educators or other health professionals able to help. Major medical centers often have diabetes education resources, as do home health nursing agencies and nurses from many state departments of health.

Many families of young children with diabetes rely solely on family members. This works well if your family is ready, reliable, able to learn, and willing to give you their time. However, for a variety of reasons, family members may not be your best choice for regular baby-sitters. One father commented, "If anyone says, 'I'd like to learn how to do diabetes care,' accept! Things happen and a neighbor or friend who understands the basics is a life saver." Competent baby-sitters can frequently be found through local diabetes organizations. Sometimes the sibling of a child with diabetes or a teen who has diabetes is quite knowledgeable about diabetes care. Diabetes camp counselors, nursing students, or intergenerational agencies also may turn up folks eager and willing to learn to care for your child. The key to finding peace and security in the knowledge that those helping you are well equipped to do so, is in their education.

Diabetes education is extremely important for anyone caring for a young child with diabetes. Signs of hypoglycemia might otherwise go unnoticed and be unattended. Very young children can't speak for themselves and the adults caring for them must know about diabetes and its treatment. Food quantities, types of foods, and timing of meals and snacks are important for caretakers to understand. In most cases, diabetes treatment centers can provide education to others at your request. In some cases, there may even be established programs already set up for this purpose.

While you are taking care of everyone else, don't forget to include yourself. Dealing with diabetes in a youngster is a major undertaking even in the best of situations. Unfortunately, most of us do not live our lives in a blissful bubble. Sometimes the stress of dealing with a chronic illness such as diabetes can be the proverbial straw that breaks the camel's back. When things aren't going well in your marriage, job, or personal life, the added stress of managing diabetes in your young child might cause you not to cope very well. Finding a family counselor, member of the clergy, or therapist may help you stay on track and give you the strength and energy you need to deal with it all.

Be a parent...not a pancreas

Pediatric diabetologist David Finegold often tells parents to "be a parent, not a pancreas." Parents often laugh at this reminder that their job is to be either mom or dad instead of the organ that does all of the diabetes regulations. Sometimes, it is easy for parents to get caught up in all of the numbers, schedules, feedings, shots, and pricks. You can't see the forest for the trees, and lose sight of your real job, which is to try to put the whole thing in balance to meet the physical, mental, and emotional needs of your child. Mothers can be very effective at being mothers but are unlikely to succeed at keeping every glucose between 100 and 200 mg/dl.

Catherine Belles, a parent, says it well. "Try not to concentrate on individual high or low readings, allowing yourself to become frustrated with them. The overall picture is most important. Take diabetes one day at a time."

Finding time together

It is well known that when there are already stresses and strains in a marriage, having a child with a chronic illness can add an unbearable stress to the relationship. Therefore, it is important to try to protect marriage and relationships by continuing to nurture them even when something like diabetes happens to your child. You may need to make a conscious effort to have fun together and make intimacy important in your relationship. Usually, fatigue, stress, and tension cause relaxed moments to become few and far between. Intimate moments for talk, quiet time together, and sexuality can suffer. Sometimes in today's culture these times actually have to be scheduled!

Parents of children with diabetes, like parents of children with other illnesses, will frequently take baby into their bed. This can happen for a variety of reasons, but it is usually out of fear of hypoglycemia or some other problem that may occur during the night. Your child enjoys the closeness of this arrangement, and it is perhaps more easy for you to fall asleep with your child nearby. However, developmental specialists do not usually recommend this practice, as it can cause separation problems at a later date.

Babies can become used to your presence and not be able to sleep otherwise. And as a parent, you may lose confidence that you will be able to tend to or care for your child if he or she is not by your side. Intimate moments between parents are limited, and baby becomes accustomed to the situation. This can create a dependency that is frequently not a healthy one for either you or your child and can be hard to break when he or she is older. In spite of the fact that sleeping with your child can save some sleep in the short term, it most likely will cause you and your child distressing sleeplessness in the long term.

The family as a whole

Since families function as a system, when one child has diabetes, the whole family is affected. Sometimes sibling relationships are as important, if not more important, as those with parents. In early childhood, siblings often spend as much time with each other as with the parent. So it is useful to understand how things might change within the family, and again consider heading off problems before they develop.

In an illness like diabetes, which affects almost every part of life, there can't help but be changes in focus and priorities. The time and effort that parents need to care for the child and to adjust emotionally may be great, and may cause other brothers or sisters to feel invisible or resentful. One mother commented, "Because Sean's presence dominated everything, there was not real time for myself." Other children in the family can become confused by these changes, and ultimately jealous. It is not surprising, due to the attention and concern of parents for the child with diabetes, that other children would feel anxious, fearful, resentful, or neglected. Parents need to be aware of these feelings.

When a child is hospitalized, brothers and sisters often fear that they did something to cause the illness. They can be frightened by the appearance of a sick sibling, and may fear that the child may die. When siblings fight, they have angry thoughts toward each other. When the brother or sister develops diabetes, they commonly think that their angry thoughts caused the diabetes. Parents and other adults can help by talking about feelings and fears, and when possible, should include the children in any education sessions for the family.

As your family adjusts over time, there may be an ongoing need to change family patterns, schedules, or leisure activities. It can become quite challenging to balance the schedules of diabetes care with an active family. One mother of four put it this way. "There are many issues with siblings that worry parents. It would almost be a luxury to only have to worry about the child with diabetes. I need to keep life moving forward on a regular schedule, which means car trips, outings, travel, and the mundane...McDonald's, grocery store, play dates, and preschool. When John was first diagnosed, it seemed like a huge deal to get out the door prepared for all contingencies."

Tips for helping brothers and sisters
Include your children in any educational sessions. Nutrition awareness is especially important, so that brothers and sisters do not unwittingly sabotage your efforts.

Talk with your children about their feelings about diabetes, and about changes that may have taken place in the family.

Reassure them that the diagnosis of diabetes was not their fault.

Help your children express fears and anxiety through conversation, drawings, and play opportunities.

Include them when possible in some caretaking responsibilities of the child with diabetes, such as preparing snacks or assisting with monitoring. Praise them for their willingness to help.

Recognize that brothers and sisters can be good at watching for signs of hypoglycemia.

As much as possible, try to spend at least a small amount of time alone with each child each day.

How Young Children Are Different

FOR THE PURPOSE OF THIS BOOK we will define the ages of children we are talking about:

INFANT: birth to 2 years. During this period, newborns will learn to sit, crawl, stand, and walk; socialize; feed themselves; wash and dry hands; put on clothing; name pictures and body parts; combine words; and throw and kick a ball.

TODDLER: age 2 to 3 years. At this age children are very busy getting into everything and exploring. They can put on a T-shirt, name things, have understandable speech, and try hard to assert their independence.

PRESCHOOLER: age 3 to 5 years. Children of this age are able to be social, dress themselves without help, play games, draw, and have understandable speech.

The developmental stages of each group are a bit arbitrary since children may be very advanced, very delayed, or most commonly, a mixture of both. However, there are definite characteristics of each stage of development that you can expect. For example, most parents are quite familiar with the "terrible twos." This is the age where "No!" is the answer to everything, even when children mean yes, as they learn to identify themselves as separate people. It is a normal process that usually occurs around age 2, yet it can be quite normal for kids to go through this "terrible" time at age 3 instead of at 2. Characteristics of these stages are discussed later in chapters 5, 6, and 7.

Size and growth

Growth during the first few years of life is at the greatest rate in a lifetime. Normal growing progresses rapidly and predictably, although it may happen in spurts. Muscle development proceeds from large muscle groups to fine motor skills. As babies grow in strength and coordination, they will go from kicking and waving arms to purposeful reaching, rolling over, sitting, crawling, and finally walking.

The brain and nerves (the central nervous system) mature quickly and depend on a constant supply of glucose in order to function well. Therefore, small frequent feedings from breast milk or formula are important to maintain the steady supply of glucose. Breast-fed babies have some ability to fight illness from antibodies they get in their mother's milk. An immature immune system leaves young children prone to colds and common childhood illnesses.

Because little children have small bodies, they have a higher risk of becoming seriously ill when problems do occur. During illness, young children can lose a large amount of fluid through the skin because of sweating. Infants are then more susceptible to dehydration than older children.

In addition, the body is made up of about 70 percent water, by weight. Babies have a higher percentage of water in their bodies than adults, and need to drink a lot of fluids. Also, infants cannot drink a large volume of fluid at one time. Fluctuations in a baby's state of hydration are quite noticeable because of their small size. Babies and young children can become dehydrated very quickly when they are ill. This can make them especially vulnerable when illness, vomiting, or diarrhea occurs. (See page 69 for a description of signs of dehydration and Chapter 4 on illness.)

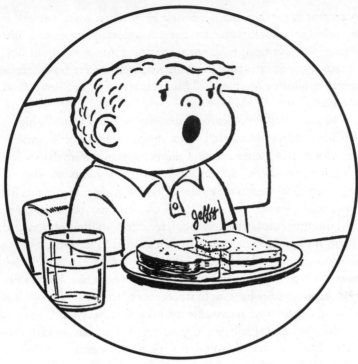

"I can't eat any more. I'm saving my crusts for the birds."

How little ones eat

Most infants nurse or eat in similar ways. In the first two years of life, a baby will move from breast or bottle feeding to drinking from a cup. The baby will learn to eat solid food from a spoon at regular meal and snack times.

In general, growth is rapid, so that even for a small body weight, little children require a relatively large number of calories. However, because their stomachs are small, they can't eat or digest very much at one time. Small, frequent feedings are important. Those who have fed hungry infants may know what happens when they drink too much milk—it often comes pouring right back out when baby burps or bends! Also, anyone who has tried to nurse an unwilling infant knows that the adult will not win the battle. When infants are not hungry, you may as well give up, because you will rarely get them to drink or eat if they don't want to. Baby will close the lips tightly, turn the head, and go to sleep when enough is enough. This is a self-protective, natural instinct. (How many adults wish a well-developed food refusal mechanism was still built in?!) In fact, when parents are persistent in fighting the battle, the scene moves to another level as the child matures. It is not just a food battle; it becomes a battle of wills.

The appetite of a toddler or preschool-age child is normally highly variable and erratic as rapid growth slows. Feeding a picky toddler can become a challenge at best. Calorie needs vary from day to day, based on wakefulness, activity, and probably a variety of other issues. Little ones like to explore, and food provides a prime area for exploration. Sometimes they'd rather play with the food than eat it. Learning the consistency, shape, size, smell, spilling power, and squish-ability of a wide variety of foods is part of learning.

Another reason that young children must eat often is that they have a limited ability to store food in reserve for a later hungry period. Adults usually have fat in storage for a "rainy day" in addition to being able to store reasonable quantities of glycogen.

Glycogen, or animal starch, is where the body stores carbohydrate for future use. We can call upon it when we are hungry, when blood glucose levels drop, or when our muscles are hard at work. It is then broken down into sugar as we need it. Babies usually have limited fat storage, and likewise have limited glycogen stores. Therefore, they cannot go without food for a very long period of time. This is why, three or four hours after feeding, baby will cry for more food, and why toddlers and young children do best with frequent small meals and snacks.

Sleep/activity

Infants need significant amounts of sleep and go from sleeping only a few hours at a time to sleeping through the night. As muscles grow and baby becomes more physically active and vigorous, it is typical to have bursts of energy and activity. After activity, toddlers usually need daily naps, with many napping heavily in both the morning and afternoon.

CHAPTER 3

Diabetes Issues in Young Children

OUR UNDERSTANDING OF HOW to care for diabetes is evolving and has changed rapidly in some areas due to improved technology, research, and new product development. One of the most significant research studies in recent years is well known as the Diabetes Control and Complications Trial or DCCT. This study, which ended in 1993, was done in fourteen centers throughout the United States and Canada on adults and teens with Type 1 diabetes. Its purpose was to determine if tight control of blood glucose levels would prevent or delay complications of diabetes. The results showed that by maintaining close to normal average blood glucose levels, complications of diabetes in adults and teens can be delayed or avoided. The problem is that we cannot take the results of this study and apply them generally to children, especially young children, because they were not studied.

Therefore, to date, there is no agreement from the experts about what the blood glucose goals should be for children. Experts do agree that goals for each child need to be based on their age, ability of the adult to care for that child, and their history of hypoglycemic events. And there are generally accepted ways of managing diabetes in a young child, based on what was learned from the DCCT study and adapted to experience with diabetes in young children. (For more, see Chapter 4, "Diabetes Control.")

First of all, all children with diabetes require insulin to grow, to develop, and to avoid high blood glucose levels. They also need a certain number of calories to grow, to develop, and to balance the insulin that is taken. The best way for parents to know how well the insulin, activity, and food are balancing is to do frequent blood glucose monitoring. The numbers from monitoring blood glucose are the tools for understanding what direction to go in managing diabetes so that low and high blood glucose levels can be avoided.

About insulin

There are a variety of different kinds of insulin products on the market today. It is wonderful to have choices, but sometimes having too many options makes things confusing. One important idea to remember is that there aren't clear right and wrong ways of treating young children with diabetes. There are, however, conservative and aggressive approaches, but the bottom line is that you and your physician will discover what works well for your child. You will know how well the insulin works from the blood glucose monitoring you do, as well as from symptoms of high and low blood glucose. Many pediatric diabetes specialists are quite conservative in their approach to treating very young children with diabetes. There are certainly risks of hypoglycemia involved that should be avoided. (See Chapter 4.)

Children, especially young children, usually take a long-acting insulin such as NPH, Lente, or Ultralente. This insulin, which provides a constant release of insulin over a long period of time, is usually taken twice, in the morning and in the evening (see graphs on the next page). These graphs show the way insulin works over time by showing when insulin works hardest and how long it lasts. You can see that there are big differences in different types of insulin. Human insulin is used most often, although some centers use pork insulin in children because it appears to provide a longer duration of action than human insulin.

Depending on the need, young children may also take a fast-acting insulin such as Humalog or Regular on a routine basis or when blood glucose levels are high. Humalog can be taken after you see how much a child actually does eat. This insulin begins to work within ten minutes after taking it and was designed to cover meals and snacks. Many young children do not require Regular or Humalog to cover their meals.

Little children can be very sensitive to even small insulin changes, and therefore it becomes necessary to sometimes adjust insulin doses by half-units. Measuring by half-units can be tricky, because not all syringes measure in half-unit increments. Measuring in half-units is

I. THREE INJECTIONS OF HUMAN NPH AND REGULAR INSULIN

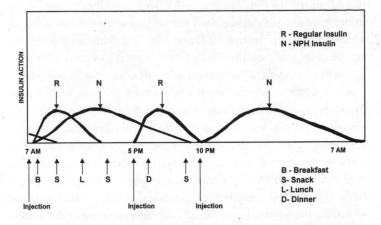

R - Regular Insulin
N - NPH Insulin

B - Breakfast
S- Snack
L- Lunch
D- Dinner

2. TWO INJECTIONS OF HUMAN NPH INSULIN

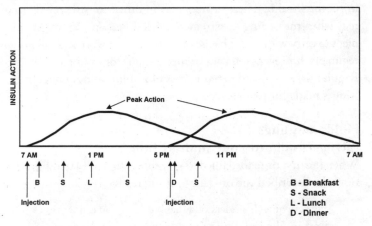

Peak Action

B - Breakfast
S - Snack
L - Lunch
D - Dinner

3. THREE INJECTIONS OF HUMAN NPH AND/OR HUMALOG INSULIN

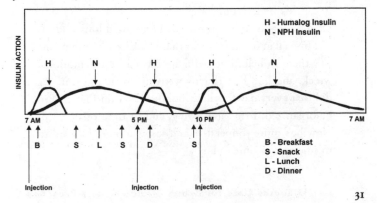

H - Humalog Insulin
N - NPH Insulin

B - Breakfast
S - Snack
L - Lunch
D - Dinner

more likely to be accurate when one person always does the "drawing up" of the insulin. There is more variability when many people draw up and inject the insulin. There are a few centers that still recommend diluting the insulin for very small children so the volume can be more easily measured. However, there is a potential for error in the process of diluting insulin, and doses may not be accurate.

Do not ever dilute insulin on your own. Dilution should be done by a pharmacist with the proper diluent, the solution made by the insulin manufacturer for your particular kind of insulin. This procedure is not done much today due to the risk of inaccuracy or errors.

Newer to the market today are insulin pens, one of which can also deliver insulin in half-unit increments. This is a device that looks like a pen that has a disposable needle on the end. A small cartridge of insulin fits inside. There is a dial so that you can set the number of units of insulin that you want, and push down on a button to inject the insulin. These devices may improve consistency of accuracy when measuring in extremely small doses, and are very convenient to carry with you. The use of a pen may not work with all insulin regimens, however. You cannot mix insulin (for example NPH and Regular) in a pen, and certain types of insulin do not come in cartridges made for pen use.

Holds and hugs
(giving insulin to your squirmy little one)

When it came time for Janice to give three-year-old Jared his injection, she described the ordeal of getting ready.

> He very quickly understood that breakfast and dinner times were insulin shot times. Jared would stand in the door and watch me and when he'd see me move toward the refrigerator door to get insulin, he'd take off like a bullet and hide under his bed. What a fight! I'd have to drag him out, screaming and crying, try to calm him, hold him, and inject him all at one time. It was a little easier when someone was there to help, but awful at best. I'd be an emotional wreck, and he'd be wringing wet with sweat and fear. We did that every day for three months. Later on I learned to be organized, firm, and loving, and in time this passed. Now he's quite cooperative and seems to look forward to this being our time to hug!

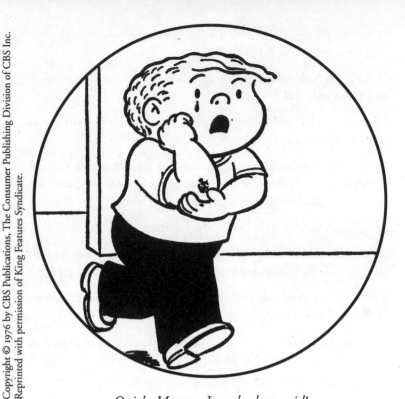

Quick, Mommy I need a bang-aid!

Helpful hints at injection times

Be as organized as possible.

Try not to draw up the insulin in front of your child. Prepare your syringe before you approach your child. Better yet, if possible, explain what you are going to do without letting the child actually see the needle. "I'm going to give your insulin now. Here comes a little pinch."

Keep everything together and have it ready to go before you get the child. For example, have the finger pricking device loaded, strip ready to go, and syringe prepared.

Don't use the word *shot* for *injection*. Children can confuse it with the shot of a gun.

Have one particular chair or area where you do injections. That makes the rest of the house "safe."

Make bed a "safe" area, which is injection free. Otherwise children may think they will be "stuck" while they sleep.

Be patient, calm, and loving, yet firm. There are no options about having the injection.

Allow your child to feel some control over the situation by allowing some choices when possible. This works best for children over two years. "Shall we give insulin here or there?"

Be quick. Anticipation is sometimes harder than the prick.

Help your child to hold still by holding the child in a hug or special way. (See the following pages for some of the holds you may use.)

Reassure your child that he has been good and that you love him. He will learn that insulin is not a punishment for bad behavior.

Tell your child that you are sorry if the insulin pinches a bit, but that she must have insulin to be healthy.

Find a second person to help hold when possible.

Be generous with hugs, love, and praise after injections. Even if your child struggles or squirms, give positive feedback on something done well.

Experience what it feels like to have an injection by injecting yourself with sterile saline, or with the syringe alone. When you discover how little discomfort there really is, it can reduce your anxiety and fear.

It can be helpful for your child to see other children with diabetes get their injections in a matter-of-fact way. Older children can be great role models for little ones.

Stickers and star charts are fun and motivating rewards for preschoolers who hold still for injections or finger pricks.

Colorful bandages can work wonders to "cover up the hole" in the skin for kids ages three to five years.

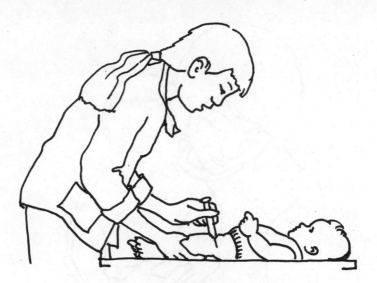

Infant "hold" for leg injection
with baby on a bed or table.

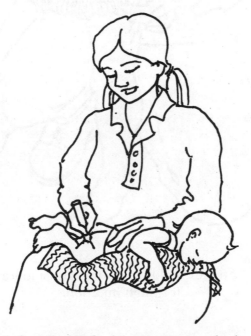

Infant "hold" for leg injection in thigh
with baby on your lap.

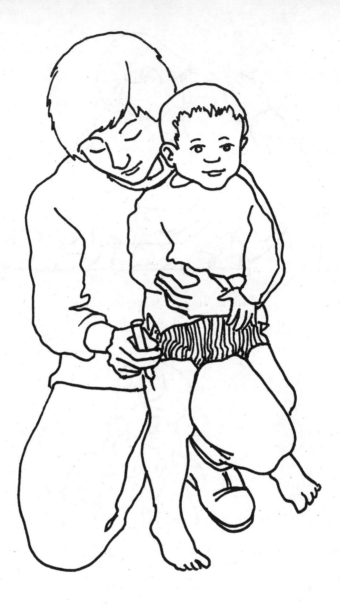

"Straddle hold" to restrain arm and leg
for thigh injection.

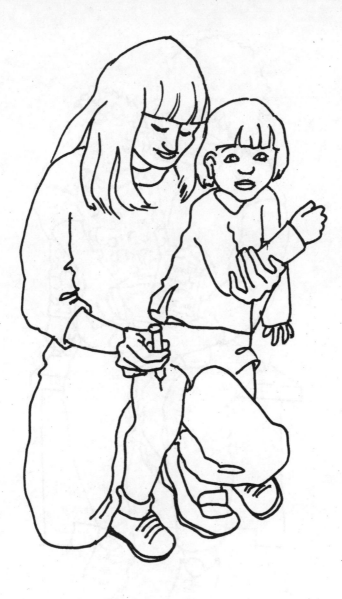

Straddle hold, similar to previous hold,
but showing another way to restrain arms

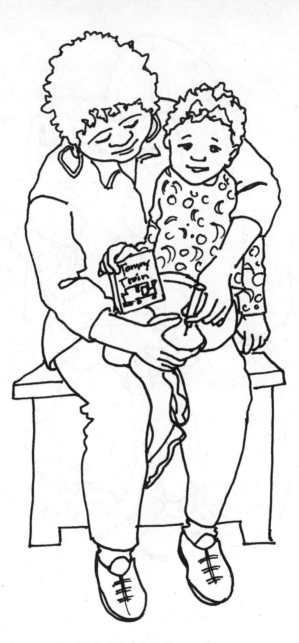

Thigh injection for toddler,
showing leg and arm restraint.

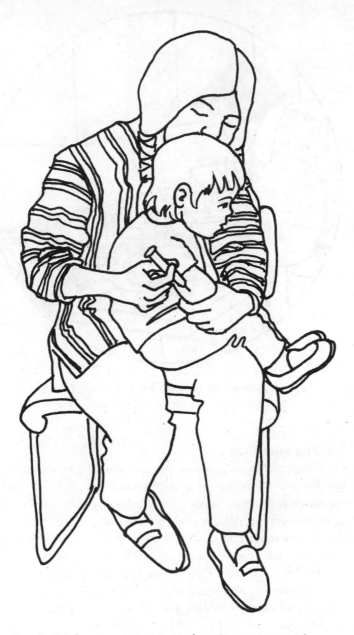

Lap hold for arm injection, showing arm restraint.

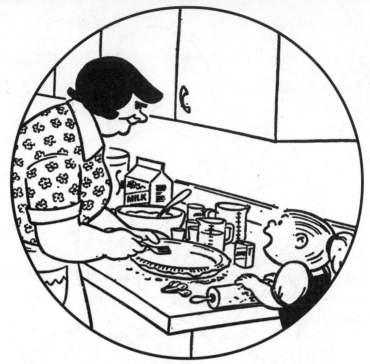

"This is a hard way to make pumpkin pie, Grandma.
Don't you know how to make the frozen kind?"

Feeding your little one

Of all the concerns parents have over their child with diabetes, probably the most frustrating yet important ones surround food. Part of the reason is that food issues go on all day, every day, and require constant attention. Also, as a cornerstone of diabetes management, there is not much that can affect blood glucose levels more than eating too much, too little, or the wrong types of foods. You can try very hard to do all of the right things, and yet blood glucose results are not where you want them to be. Studies have shown that parents feel guilty and worry a lot about food issues. You may live with constant questions, such as "Did I feed him enough?" "Did I feed him too much?" "Since he never ate pizza before, I wonder how it will affect blood glucose." "Do I have the right foods prepared?" "Am I running late for my meal schedule?" "Am I a bad parent because I said No to the candy?" "Is it OK that I or his sister eat something that is not on John's meal plan?" "How do I make him eat if he's not hungry?" These and other questions are real issues, and for the most part, there aren't any perfect solutions. Doing the best you can doesn't always feel good enough.

One of the cornerstones of treating diabetes is now called Medical Nutrition Therapy or MNT. The aim of MNT is to give your child enough calories to grow and gain weight, to balance insulin peaks and activity, to avoid a high or low blood glucose, and to keep the child healthy. Young children should grow completely normally, but it is important to check height and weight at three-month intervals and even more often with a young infant. Weight and height increases help to show that baby is getting enough calories and using the calories that are eaten. If blood glucose control runs very high, the child can lose calories in the urine and may not gain weight!

When your child has diabetes, one of the team members who meets with you is a registered dietitian who will consider your child's eating pattern. The nutrition plan that you are given should reflect your baby's and your family's individual eating habits, the kind of insulin being used, and how many calories are needed. At first, your child may be extremely hungry, and this pattern may continue until the child regains any weight lost. The meal plan is usually adjusted quickly when more normal eating patterns return, and then at regular intervals as your child grows.

Infants may require a frequent feeding schedule, and toddlers and preschool age children usually need at least three meals and three snacks a day. The snacks usually fall at mid-morning, mid-afternoon, and before bedtime. The goal is to have a steady supply of carbohydrates to balance insulin needs. Sometimes extra snacks may be necessary.

There are a number of types of MNT plans currently being used. Most commonly, people are using either a system of carbohydrate (carb) counting, or an exchange system, or sometimes a merger of both. With the carb counting plan, a certain number of grams of carbohydrates is given at each meal and snack. For example, Frankie may take in 45 grams in cereal and milk at breakfast, 3 P.M., and 11 P.M., and only 10 grams in between when he has only a bottle. The food exchange system places foods into six groups and has a plan for what number of "exchanges" or servings you should use from each group for each meal and snack.

For an infant, much will depend on whether or not the infant is bottle or breast-fed, the type of formula used, whether the infant eats solid food, how well the infant eats, and whether meal times are on a schedule. Infants may require feedings at four-hour intervals all day and night. When baby is able to sleep longer during the night, your doctor, diabetes nurse educator, or dietitian will help suggest changes in food or insulin to make sure things are balanced. For example, giving baby cereal with the last feeding of the night may allow the baby to sleep longer without having hypoglycemia at night.

When to wean

If baby is breast-feeding at the time of diagnosis, try to continue to do so. There is enough disruption of normal family schedules and other family stress that to cause any more changes by trying to wean from the breast during this time is usually not a good idea. Breast-feeding has many advantages for both mother and baby. However, when baby has diabetes, the hard part of breast-feeding is in not knowing how much milk the baby has taken. If you have six ounces of milk in a bottle and the baby takes three ounces, you can see what is left and might consider checking blood sugar early or trying some additional calories before the next feeding. But when baby is breast-feeding it is hard to know for sure how much has actually been consumed. In spite of this, it is worth the effort to try to breast-feed up until twelve months, with consideration given to supplementing with a bottle. Pumping breast milk and freezing or storing it for another time helps to solve the problem somewhat, plus allows dad or another adult to help. During this time, extra blood glucose monitoring will be important along with nighttime blood checks.

Starting solids foods

At age four to six months, most infants begin to learn to swallow solid foods by starting with rice cereal at the time of one of their feedings. As the baby grows and develops the muscles and ability to swallow better, semi-solid foods are added to the plan. The progression usually includes a variety of types of cereals, fruits, fruit juices, vegetables, meats, and eggs. You will most likely follow a plan suggested by your pediatrician and modified by a dietitian to balance insulin regimens.

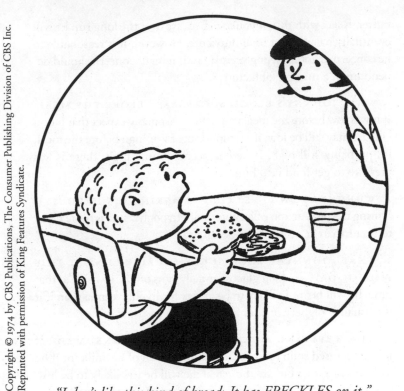

"I don't like this kind of bread. It has FRECKLES on it."

Finicky eaters

Although the development of Humalog insulin has helped to solve
the "kid-won't-eat" problem, one difficulty parents still face from time
to time is the battle of food. You know that Johnny had his insulin
and that it will be peaking soon. You know that he squashed his lunch
sandwich and threw it on the floor, and pinched all his grapes between his forefinger and thumb! You know that he should be eating well-balanced meals for good nutrition and health. You know
that this is normal kid stuff, the way most toddlers eat. You also
know that he may become hypoglycemic because he didn't eat
enough food to cover the insulin. So now what do you do?

First of all, it is normal for children to eat sporadically. Appetites
are usually not consistent and can vary from one time of day to another, and from one day to the next. Johnny may eat nothing but
bananas and yogurt for two weeks then switch to peaches and peanut

butter. Relax with this, if you can, because over the long run he will eventually balance out total nutrients. However, it is reasonable to be concerned about hypoglycemia. Your level of concern should depend upon a number of factors:

1. WHAT JOHNNY'S BLOOD SUGAR WAS BEFORE THE MEAL. If it was low before the meal you could reasonably expect that blood glucose may still be low; if his blood sugar was high before the meal, it's probably still high. If he has been running high, there is less pressure to get food into him.

2. WHEN INSULIN IS PEAKING (WORKING ITS HARDEST). During the peak action of insulin times, hypoglycemia is more likely to occur than at other times. See graph 2.

3. WHAT JOHNNY'S BLOOD SUGAR USUALLY RUNS AT THIS TIME OF DAY. If blood glucose usually runs on the low side at that time, he will be more likely to be at risk for hypoglycemia than if it is a usually "higher" time of day.

4. THE TYPE AND QUANTITY OF FOOD CONSUMED. If Johnny refused solid food but at least drank all of his milk, or if he refused vegetables but ate the cereal, he will be less likely to be low.

5. THE TIME OF THE NEXT BOTTLE, MEAL, OR SNACK. If he refuses food but you know that he has a snack coming up shortly, you can be less concerned than if he has to get through the night without food.

As hard as it is to do frequent finger pricks to determine blood glucose numbers, this is one way to help you decide your course of action. If blood glucose is on the low side of normal, (<100 mg/dl or 5.5 mmoles) you will probably want to make an effort to try to get some food or drink into Johnny.

If he refuses regular meals or snacks, try these foods: fruit juice, whole milk, yogurt, Popsicle, applesauce, crackers, or plain cookies. Sometimes you may need to be creative in your approach. One mom reported that when eighteen-month-old Jodi was being temperamental and wouldn't eat, she would set three M&M's out on the table. Jodi would fuss around and cry but eventually pick up one M&M and eat it, then the next. Only then could her mother get her to drink something that had carbohydrates in it.

Robby's mother says, "Robby loves to look at photographs, especially of himself. At meals and snacks, I would say, 'Eat a cracker and I'll show you another picture.' He would become very animated with this game and it worked wonders. It worked best when he was fourteen to fifteen months."

Another parent tells of another food tip:

> When Sam won't eat, I like to try to get him to eat a Nite Bite bar (a bar that has 15 grams carbohydrate, which includes cornstarch, for sticking power). But usually he won't eat that unless I break it up into little pieces and let him dip each bite in whipped topping. That's the only way I can get it into him.

The mother of three-year-old John said:

> I usually try to save things that I know John really likes and will easily take for when he is low. We save juice boxes for this purpose. Another food that works is little cookie sticks that come in a package with sparkle icing. This is magic…it works out to be one bread and one fat exchange. Also, John has started to make the "I feel low—I need juice—I feel better" connection!

Giving special sweet treats to treat hypoglycemia is fine in young children to encourage them to eat. However, be guarded about this practice because as children get older, they may learn that if they don't eat, they get candy later.

Extra-Light Snacks

Approximately 10 grams of carbohydrate per serving

FOOD	SERVING SIZE
Banana	1/4 of 1 large banana
Graham crackers	2 squares
Applesauce (unsweetened)	1/3 cup (or Mott's snack cup)
Arrowroot cookie	2 cookies
Cheerios	2/3 cup
Cheese Nips (Nabisco)*	13
Cheez-its (Sunshine)*	17
Goldfish crackers (Pepperidge Farm)*	28 pieces
Club crackers (Keebler)*	5
Town House crackers (Keebler)*	5
Oysterettes (Nabisco, Sunshine)	18
Animal crackers	7
Animal crackers* (R.W. Frookie)	6
Kix cereal	2/3 cup
Jell-O fruit bar	1
Wheat Thins (Nabisco)*	9
Sherbet	1/4 cup
Frozen mini waffles with light syrup* (Eggo minis)	2 waffles, 1 tsp. syrup
Fruit Roll-ups (General Mills)	1
Pretzel logs (Nabisco)	4
Raisins	1 tbsp. or 1/2 ounce
Popcorn	2 cups
Apricot, fresh	3 small to medium
Green pepper, fresh	2 cups
Broccoli, fresh or cooked	1 large stalk (2 cups)
Bread stick (Stella D'oro)	1 1/2
Carrot	2
Tea biscuit (Social)*	2
Ritz Bits (Cheese)*	9
Ritz Bits (peanut butter)*	7
Life Saver Flavor Pops (frozen)†	1 pop
Bite-size Pecan Sandies (Keebler)*	4
Dannon Frozen Yogurt on a Stick†	1 pop

*Has an added fat serving

†Not recommended for toddlers

Extra-Light Snacks (continued)

FOOD	SERVING SIZE
Apple†	3/4 of small apple
Saltines	4
Frozen low-fat yogurt	1/4 cup
Sugar-free pudding	1/3 cup

Light Snacks

15 grams of carbohydrate per serving

FOOD	SERVING SIZE
Triscuit crackers (Nabisco)*	6 crackers
Goldfish crackers (Pepperidge Farm)*	45 crackers
Cheez-its (Sunshine)*	29
Cheese Nips (Nabisco)*	20
Oyster crackers, small	60
Oysterettes, large (Nabisco, Sunshine)	30
Animal crackers	7
Cinnamon raisin English muffin	1 muffin
English muffin	1/2 muffin
Cantaloupe	1/3 medium melon or 1 cup cubes
Grapes	15 small
Orange	1
Apple	1 small
Banana	1/2 (4 oz.)
Kix cereal (General Mills)	1 cup
Fruit cocktail (canned, water pack)	1/2 cup
Combos*	1 oz.
Cinnamon raisin bread	1 slice
Ginger snaps (Nabisco)	3
Chocolate snaps (Nabisco)	3
Nilla wafers*	5
Applesauce, unsweetened	1/2 cup
Corn chips*	1 ounce (2/3 cup)
Green pea Cup-a-Soup (Lipton) with saltines	1 packet, 2 crackers

*Has an added fat serving

†Not recommended for toddlers

Light Snacks (continued)

FOOD	SERVING SIZE
Spring vegetable Cup-a-Soup (Lipton) with Wheat thins	1 packet, 8 crackers
Wheat thins*	14
Frozen waffle (Eggo buttermilk)*	1 round
Frozen mini waffle* with light syrup	4 waffles, 1 tsp. syrup
Peach	1
Canned peaches (water pack)	1/2 cup
Popcorn, low-fat, microwave	3 cups
Honeydew	1/8 medium melon or 1 cup cubes
Thins pretzel twists	4
Cheerios	1 cup
Teddy grahams*	15
Whole wheat toast	1 slice
Ritz crackers*	8 crackers
Pizza*	1/2 slice

Medium Snacks

30 grams of carbohydrate per serving

FOOD	SERVING SIZE
Wheat Thins*	28
Ritz crackers (Nabisco)*	12
Matzoh (Goodmans)	2 6-inch squares
Lunch crackers (Nabisco)	2
Applesauce (unsweetened)	1/2 cup
Rice	2/3 cup
Lorna Doones*	12
Grapes and melba rounds	17 grapes, 8 rounds
Pretzel rods	2

FOOD	SERVING SIZE
Peach with Wheat Thins (Nabisco)*	1 medium peach, 14 Wheat Thins
Apple with Goldfish crackers (Pepperidge Farm)*	1 apple, 45 pieces

*Has an added fat serving

Medium Snacks (continued)

FOOD	SERVING SIZE
Cantaloupe with popcorn	1/3 medium melon, 3 cups popcorn
Honeydew melon with pretzels	1/8 medium melon, 4 thin pretzel twists
English muffin and raisins	1/2 muffin, 2 tbsp. raisins
Graham crackers	6 squares
Animal crackers	14

Medium Plus Snacks
35 grams of carbohydrate per serving

FOOD	SERVING SIZE
Graham crackers	6 squares
English muffin with low-sugar jam	1 muffin, 2 tsp. jam
RyKrisp crackers, apple	3 triple crackers, 1/2 apple
English muffin, with an apricot	1 muffin, 1 medium apricot
Cinnamon raisin English muffin with low-sugar jelly	1 muffin, 2 tsp. jelly
Cheerios with banana and milk	1 cup Cheerios, 1/2 small banana, 1/2 cup milk
Angel food cake	1/12 cake
Saltines and Gatorade	12 saltines, 8 oz. Gatorade
Popcorn and orange	2 cups popcorn, 1 orange
Macaroni with spray margarine	1 1/4 cups macaroni
Frozen low-fat yogurt	1 cup
Whole strawberries with vanilla yogurt	2 1/2 cups fruit, 1/2 cup yogurt
Fresh fruit (apple, peach, nectarine) and pretzels	1 piece fruit, 5 thin twists

Avoiding the short-order-cook syndrome

Are you a mom or dad who runs around chasing little Sara with food or drink, bribing, begging, cajoling, and ultimately forcing her to eat something? (Guess who will win that battle—it won't be you!) As Sara gets close to toddlerhood, the problem may get worse as she quite naturally starts to become her "own person." Children at this age begin to recognize that they are separate from everything and everyone else. That is why the age of "no" emerges at this point. It is a moment of self-definition. When these struggles begin, it is quite easy for a parent or caregiver to fall into the trap of becoming food chaser and short-order cook. Some parents admit to preparing three or more different meals in the hope that their child will eat one of them!

So, what can you do to avoid falling into the short-order-cook trap? The first step is to recognize that the trap exists and decide not to let it rule. You will need to figure out your plan of action. Then do your best to stick to it. Here are some ideas.

Always keep foods on hand that your child likes and is most likely to eat.

When possible, provide a choice of two items. "Do you want a bologna or cheese sandwich?" Decide that one alternative choice is enough and stick to it. Children will learn that they can choose "A" or "B" but there are no other options.

Eat what your child eats. Set a good example for your child when you are eating.

Let your child feed himself, because children can and do regulate their own calories and nutrition.

Keep on hand at least one easily served alternative, especially when you are introducing new foods. (For example, on the day you decide to see how Johnny does with noodle casserole, you may want to keep a peanut butter sandwich on standby.)

Keep mealtime pleasant and relaxed. Try to avoid the unpleasant battles that can occur over eating.

Allow your child to help in preparing the meal. Children are more likely to eat something they made themselves.

Introduce a new food along with well-liked foods, and introduce it early in the meal.

Ask your doctor about a flexible insulin regimen that will allow you to better match insulin to the food consumed. (See page 30 for more on Humalog.)

Set a time limit at the table. Encourage your child to drink milk or juice if the child doesn't eat.

Holidays and special occasions

Parents and teachers of preschoolers generally have the difficult task of providing safe, fun, and creative learning situations for their children. Yet, as most parents can testify, children have a short attention span. The task of keeping a child this age happily occupied can be challenging. Children with diabetes have a more difficult time because many activities and parties center around food, especially sweets. Preschool-age children can have difficulty understanding why they are denied what others can eat. Educating school staff about special occasion foods and learning how to fit some sweet foods into the meal plan can help children have fun without swerving too far off course in their diabetes plan. A bit of advance planning can help the child feel part of the group, yet not compromise diabetes control.

Talk with staff at the preschool to come up with a plan about how to handle snacks and parties. Then write down the plan so everyone will know about it. If agreeable to those concerned, sometimes a note to other parents stating that there is a child with diabetes in the program can be helpful in encouraging other parents to send healthy snacks instead of sweets.

Tips for special occasions

Send a list of acceptable special occasion foods to your center.

Keep a supply of acceptable foods at the center in case there are sweet treats offered that you do not want your child to have. Nonperishables might include a can of diet soda, crackers, plain cookies, fruit roll-ups, dried fruit, nuts, or popcorn. Don't forget to check and restock the supply regularly.

Allow your child a small portion of what is being served, such as cake without the icing, or ice cream without the cake.

Fill an Easter basket with treats other than food, such as coloring books, pencils, or stickers.

On Halloween, trade your child's bag of treats for something special the child has been wanting. In some cases neighbors will hand out special treats for your child with diabetes, such as sugar-free gum, raisins, crackers, or stickers.

Ask the school to notify you in advance when they know a special party will be held so that you can plan insulin doses. By the same token, if a party spontaneously springs up, the staff should notify you that blood glucose levels may be altered that day because of special food.

Monitoring and record keeping

Monitoring blood glucose and urine ketones are important to do in young children with diabetes. Testing your child's blood glucose may be the single most important thing you can do to help to manage diabetes and give direction to your child's care. Frequent blood glucose monitoring will help to give you peace of mind that blood glucose levels are running well, or point you in the right direction in knowing what to do if they aren't. It is not just doing the test that makes the difference but how you use the test results.

Eventually you will learn to look for patterns of high or low blood glucose. For this reason, it is important to keep daily records of your child's blood glucose, schedule, insulin, and any extraordinary events that may happen. For example, sickness, being off-schedule, not eating, eating a lot, or eating special occasion foods at a birthday party are all important comments to record. The patterns will help you and your health care team to determine if any changes need to be made in food, insulin doses, or scheduling.

Blood glucose monitoring

Sometimes parents comment that pricking little fingers and toes is one of the hardest parts of diabetes management for them. Of course, part of the problem is directly due to how difficult the pricks are for each individual child. Some youngsters will act out more than others, and not necessarily due to discomfort; it is just the idea of the whole thing. However, if that is the case, as for injections, these tips may be helpful.

Fingertips, toes, and the outer part of the heel in very young children are good places to use. Some people have also suggested the earlobe for little kids, but the earlobe is seldom used.

For very tiny fingers, you will need to find a very gentle finger-prick device, and learn to press it hard enough against the skin to get enough blood, but not so hard that it goes very deep. There are finger-pricking devices that have an adjustable depth of needle penetration, which is ideal for little children with tiny and sensitive fingers.

Take care not to use the center part of the heel for pricks because repeated pokes in that site have been associated with bone infections.

Explain everything you do, and why you are doing it. Even babies too small to talk or understand will be reassured by your voice, and as one mother put it, "They catch on quick, and in return, can help you."

Be alert for any skin breakdown where you prick, and try to rotate sites as much as possible.

Alcohol is not necessary for cleansing as it can be very drying to baby's skin. Soap and water work best to cleanse the site. Just make sure that it is well dried.

Try to keep baby's bed a "safe" area as much as possible, the same as with injections. Pick baby up to hold or cradle him for a blood test so that he doesn't learn that he will be poked and prodded even while "safe" in his bed.

Meters
You may have a diabetes educator who will show you various types of meters and give you suggestions for testing. Things to think about when deciding what brand of meter to use for a young child are:

THE SIZE OF THE DROP OF BLOOD REQUIRED TO DO A TEST. Meters that require larger blood sample sizes will be more difficult if baby doesn't bleed well. You will then have to repeat the test or reprick fingers, heels, or toes.

METER PORTABILITY. For a very young child, it is easier to have a blood test strip or meter that can easily be taken to baby's finger or toe. Or, you may wish to use a little "pipette," which is a tube that takes the blood from the finger to carry it to the meter.

EASE OF USE. Although most meters today are quite easy to use, it will be important for you to find the type that works most easily for you.

METER APPROVED FOR NEWBORNS. There are certain meters that may not work well for newborns. Not all meters have been approved by the Food and Drug Administration (FDA) for use in newborns. Very new babies can have fetal hemoglobin, which gives an inaccurate value for certain types of meters.

Urine ketones

Ketones are the end product of burning body fat for energy. They are a "red flag" for possible danger. They may not mean anything important, or they may mean that changes need to be made quickly in your child's insulin doses. As a parent, it is not so important for you to be the one to interpret why ketones are present, but rather to report to your doctor or health care team that they are. Ketones are most likely to form:
- if there isn't enough insulin present to meet the needs of body cells
- during illness
- if your child hasn't eaten for a while (starvation can come even overnight for very young children)
- after hypoglycemia

Ideally, there will not be ketones present in the urine. However, if there are ketones, knowing the amount (small, moderate, large), along with a blood glucose number, will help your doctor or diabetes educator guide you in treatment. It is important to check for ketones if your child has a blood glucose over 300 mg/dl (16.6 mmoles), or is not feeling well.

Testing for urine ketones is done by dipping a urine strip in urine, waiting a certain amount of time (based on manufacturer's directions), and comparing the color to a chart on the bottle. When your child is in diapers, checking for ketones can be challenging. Since babies don't "pee" on demand, catching a few drops is not easy.

Current brands of diapers contain silica gel products that are very absorbent and make it difficult to squeeze out a drop of urine. Ideas for getting a few drops of urine from disposable diapers are:

Put a couple of gauze pads or cotton balls in the dry diaper in an area most likely to get wet.

Buy inexpensive diaper liners that do not contain silica gel.

Pick the wettest stuffing out of the diaper and put it into a syringe from which you have removed the needle and plunger. Then push the plunger in to try to squeeze out a drop onto the strip.

And for older kids:
- If the child is still using a potty chair, you can easily dip a urine strip in before discarding the urine.
- Ask your hospital or medical supplier for a urine collection "hat" that sits under the commode seat to collect urine.
- Or, if the child is old enough, have your child void directly on the strip.

The treatment of ketones in the urine includes:
- figuring out why they are present (not enough insulin, starvation, hypoglycemia).
- making adjustments to insulin doses.
- encouraging fluids to prevent dehydration.

CHAPTER 4

Diabetes Control

EVEN IF YOU HAVE BEEN given specific blood glucose goals to work toward from your doctor, it is common to wonder how closely you need to stick to them. Parents wonder how tightly to control blood glucose levels and what the risks are of having numbers that are too high or too low. For parents of little children, there are "educated guess" answers to these questions, but specific guidelines for blood glucose control have not been set for younger children.

Diabetes control generally is looked at in three different ways. One way is called the glycoslylated hemoglobin (HbA1c) level. This is a test done on a blood sample, and can be thought of as the average blood glucose level for the previous two months. Laboratory values usually differ from each other, but the normal value is usually less than 6.5 percent. For older children, adolescents, and adults, usually the closer you can get the HbA1c to normal without having severe or frequent hypoglycemia, the better. However, if a low HbA1c is at the expense of a lot of severe episodes of hypoglycemia, changes should be made. It is not just the average that is important, but also the consistency of the blood glucose results day in and day out.

Another way to follow diabetes control is to evaluate the daily blood glucose numbers. These numbers done usually at least four times a day in young children will give you a picture of how things are going on a daily basis. These numbers are used together with the HbA1c and urine ketone results to make treatment decisions about insulin type, frequency of injections, meal schedules, and types of foods eaten.

The third way to decide diabetes control is clinical signs. If your child has frequent or severe hypoglycemia, or often shows signs of high blood glucose (such as ketones in the urine or soaking-wet diapers), diabetes is not well controlled. Together, you and your diabetes specialist can decide how control is going. If one or more of these three areas is not going well, changes will need to be made.

It is well known that for adults and teens with diabetes, the "lower" or "tighter" diabetes control is, the better the chance of preventing or delaying complications of diabetes. In other words, for each little drop in the HbA1c level, the more kidney, heart, nerve, and eye disease can be prevented. The problem is that it is not known at what age it becomes important to tighten up control. Conversely, some studies have shown that teens with diabetes who were diagnosed before the age of six years may have some differences in the way they learn and perform, possibly due to undetected hypoglycemia at an early age. Therefore, it seems prudent and conservative to avoid hypoglycemia.

Most pediatric diabetes specialists believe that the before-meal target blood glucose range for children under six years of age should be at or around 100 to 200 mg/dl (5.5 to 11.1 mmoles). This range is set a little higher than for older children in order to prevent frequent or severe low blood glucose. This target range, however, should be based on the child's age, frequency and severity of low blood glucose episodes, and the child's ability to recognize that he or she feels lows and tell someone. You can think of this target as the bull's-eye. There will be many times that you don't hit the bull's-eye but may be quite satisfied that you even hit close to the target at all!

Hypoglycemia (low blood glucose)

When there is not enough glucose in the bloodstream, all other cells also become deprived of glucose. And when those cells happen to be brain or nerve cells, there can be signs of irritability, confusion, poor coordination, combativeness, fatigue, and sleepiness. A child may not always experience symptoms of hypoglycemia when blood glucose is low.

The immediate danger of hypoglycemia is that a rapidly falling blood glucose can make it difficult for your child to eat, drink, or swallow. Sometimes, although the child may be physically able to drink, he or she may be uncooperative and unwilling to drink or eat. If blood glucose continues to drop, unconsciousness or a seizure can develop. This is why it is important to observe and treat hypoglycemia early.

During a seizure, the brain wildly pumps out impulses that spread to the rest of the body. This can result in unresponsiveness, jerking movements of the arms and legs, urine incontinence, and an unusual cry or grunting. Obviously, this is an unhealthy situation, and should be avoided whenever possible. Fortunately, a child who has a hypoglycemic seizure that is treated promptly usually recovers well. Mild hypoglycemia does not seem to have any permanent effect, although again, research shows that some teens who have been diagnosed with diabetes before the age of five years have mild cognitive changes, possibly related to undetected low blood glucose. Severe hypoglycemia, meaning untreated unconsciousness for a prolonged period of time, can cause damage to the brain and nerves, or even death.

Since infants and young children cannot say how they feel, those caring for them must watch for signs of low blood sugar and test blood often if low blood glucose is suspected. Signs of low blood sugar in a young child can be very hard to detect. This is the part that is worrisome for most parents and caretakers. Unusual or different behaviors may be the only noticeable sign of a low blood sugar. Behavioral cues can be hard to discern from normal infant and toddler behavior.

Although the symptoms of low blood glucose come on rather quickly sometimes, it is rare for a child to have such severe symptoms that you cannot readily correct the problem. Some children, even as young as age three, are able to sense that they are "low," hungry, or don't feel good and tell someone. The important thing is to be prepared for whatever could happen. This means having supplies for treating hypoglycemia available to you all of the time and to always check unusual behavior or signs of hypoglycemia by doing a blood glucose check. If your child is showing signs of low blood glucose and you are not able to do a blood glucose test, treat for hypoglycemia anyway. If Johnny is not low, you may cause a high blood glucose for a while, but if he does have low blood glucose you will prevent it from dropping further.

An infant who is hypoglycemic may look pale or be listless, fussy, sweaty, sleepy, crying, or irritable. Toddlers and preschoolers may also be hungry, have temper tantrums, or have nightmares or restless sleep. What is tough to decide sometimes, however, is whether your child is having a typical out-of-control, kicking, fighting, two-year-old tantrum, or whether he or she is having low blood glucose. John's mom says that he "gets sort of manic, like a child trying to fight sleep." Other parents have said it seems like the child is trying to fight the symptoms of the low.

Let your glucose meter be your guide when making decisions about what to do. Check blood glucose when you are unsure about behavior. Most parents say that distinguishing between temper tantrums and hypoglycemia gets easier over time as they begin to recognize their child's usual response to low blood glucose. Making sure does require some extra pricks, but your peace of mind and security are well worth the effort.

Treat baby at the first sign of low blood glucose, whether the sign is from baby's appearance or behavior or from a low blood glucose number. Treatment for a low blood glucose in an infant is to feed the infant 5 to 10 grams of carbohydrate. You may want to try these strategies to see what will work best for your infant.

- 2 to 4 ounces of baby fruit juice or milk
- 4 ounces of 5 percent glucose water (glucose water can be found at most pharmacies)
- Dip baby's bottle nipple, pacifier, or your finger in Karo syrup if baby will not take a bottle.
- Rub cake decorator gel between baby's gum and cheek.
- CAUTION: Never use honey in infants younger than one year of age due to the risk of botulism in very young children.

For your toddler or preschool-age child:
- Offer 4 ounces of your child's favorite juice or beverage with carbohydrate.
- Follow up with 15 grams carbohydrate in crackers, cereal, or plain cookies.
- If the child is being fussy and will not drink juice and eat crackers, progress to foods with sugar that he or she may be more likely to eat, such as cake decorator gel, ice cream, raisins, candy, marshmallows, or fruit.

You may be concerned about falling into the trap of allowing your child to dictate what he or she will or won't eat, or of setting up bad habits for later on. It is wise to be aware of that possibility for years ahead. However, your immediate problem is the treatment of low blood glucose, and the answer is to do whatever it takes to get carbohydrate inside your child in the easiest and least stressful way. Force feeding is not a good idea and can create problems since young children are naturally selective about what they will and won't eat or drink.

Try to become familiar with the amount of carbohydrate in the food you use to treat hypoglycemia. Check the package for nutrient information, or ask your child's dietitian.

It is always a good idea to test blood glucose levels 15 to 20 minutes after treating hypoglycemia to make certain that the blood glucose is rising. If it is not, you will need to repeat the treatment. While you are waiting for blood glucose levels to rise, stay with your child to make sure he or she is improving. Because these times can be as scary for your child as for you, your child will probably want comforting. (You probably will, too…go for it! Closeness, holding, and hugs help!)

How to Treat Hypoglycemia in Young Children

AGE OF CHILD	AMOUNT OF CARBOHYDRATE	SAMPLE CHOICES
Infants	5–10 grams carb	• 4 oz. baby fruit juice or milk • 4 oz. of 5% glucose water • 1–2 tsp. Karo syrup • 1/2 sm. tube cake decorator gel icing on nipple, pacifier, or finger • CAUTION: Do not give honey to children under age 1
Toddlers and Pre-schoolers	5–10 grams carb	• 2 glucose tablets (break in half) • 4–6 oz. fruit juice • 4–6 oz. regular soda • 1 sm. tube cake decorator gel • and/or crackers, cookies, cereal candy (e.g. Smartees: 1 sleeve = 3 grams carb)

Glucagon

If your child refuses food or drink and blood glucose levels remain low, you will need to give an injection of glucagon. If you do not have glucagon, ask your doctor or health team about obtaining a prescription. Glucagon is a hormone that quickly raises blood glucose levels. It comes in a vial along with a syringe full of water. The water must be pushed into the vial to mix the glucagon into solution. The mixed solution is then pulled back into the syringe, ready for injection. You give glucagon if your child is hypoglycemic and not able to eat, drink, or swallow a form of carbohydrate. Never force food or beverages into a child's mouth if the child cannot swallow or is unconscious, as he or she could choke or inhale it into the lungs. For children under six years of age, it is generally recommended that if you need to give glucagon, 0.5 milligrams (or half the total dose) is probably enough. There is a 0.5 milligrams line on the syringe. There should be no harm done if you give the whole dose, but it is probably more than a young child needs and it can cause vomiting. There is no reason why glucagon should not be used in a situation where your child is profoundly hypoglycemic. The only "con" is that it can sometimes cause nausea and vomiting and high blood glucose levels afterwards. It is really important that you have glucagon in your diaper bag, purse, or pocket, so you always have it available.

Preventing hypoglycemia

Preventing hypoglycemia in a young child with diabetes is an enormous effort and should be the biggest goal in your care. Preventing high blood glucose is also important but unless there are ketones present in the urine, there is little immediate concern.

The timing of feedings, meals, and snacks should attempt to match the way insulin works. Insulin products have peak action time periods, and meals and snacks should try to match these peaks. (See Chapter 3.) When insulin and food are not in balance, a low or high blood glucose can result. Blood glucose monitoring will help you make decisions about balancing food and insulin.

Usually parents find they must adjust their schedules to meet the needs of their child, and must also adjust the child's schedule to fit in insulin injections, blood glucose monitoring, feedings, and naps.

Infants usually fall into an internal clock schedule, as they feed or sleep on demand.

In general, keeping to a schedule is useful in preventing hypoglycemia. A rule of thumb to try to keep blood glucose levels steady is to stay within an hour of your usual schedule for insulin doses, meals, snacks, activity, and naps. Obviously it is not humanly possible to attend to a rigorous schedule all of the time, and things do crop up in life. So, the goal should be to develop a flexible schedule approach, one that minimizes randomness yet allows for the interruptions of life.

It is useful to be on the lookout for daily changes in your child's eating activity and schedule, and make note of them. You might call this "anticipatory problem solving." You will need first to have a firm understanding of the way insulin, food, and activity balance each other (see Chapter 3). Once you understand this, you will be able to expect what direction blood glucose levels might go, and be prepared to make changes. For example, if Bobby always eats a great breakfast and morning snack, and isn't low before lunch, then you would not anticipate a problem. But if your child eats only half his breakfast, picks at his snack, and plays through his morning nap, then it is reasonable to think that he might be low by lunch. In that case, you may want to test blood glucose before the snack and offer juice or milk throughout the morning.

When you think about the direction of blood glucose levels, consider the type or amount of food and drink Suzy had. You might watch for differences in the effect of different types of foods or drinks on her blood glucose levels. Do blood glucose levels look different on a cereal morning than on a pancake morning? On a cereal morning, do blood glucose levels look different on a crispy rice day than on a toasted oat day? Consider spacing of meals and snacks. Are they running close together or too far apart? Is she eating or drinking between meals and snacks? Do you provide enough food or drink to cover activity? Do you give too much food or drink during an activity or in treatment of lows? How regular is your child's schedule? Are nap times regular? The more consistent the schedule, the better you can control hypoglycemic events.

Ellen Warner, a parent, comments:

> It took a few mistakes for us to learn we always had to be prepared for a low and so did the preschool teacher, baby-

sitter, and grandparents. Make sure that you always have something like glucose tablets, icing, or Smartees. The lows come at the worst times and you're never home. We keep stuff in the glove compartment in the car. I always have something in my pocket when we go on a walk. Always!

These are not easy problems and there aren't always easy solutions. Learning as much as you can about managing diabetes, calling your diabetes specialist frequently for questions and concerns, being prepared for hypoglycemia by carrying supplies, doing frequent monitoring, and educating others are important strategies.

Things to pack in a purse or diaper bag

FOR SHORT OUTING (LESS THAN TWO HOURS): meter, strips, lancets; juice box, cake gel, crackers, glucagon; alcohol wipes if not near water

FOR HALF-DAY OUTING: supplies for short outing plus extra snacks, insulin, and syringes if over a meal

FOR DAYLONG OR OVERNIGHT OUTING: above listed supplies plus urine ketone strips

FOR LONGER TRIPS: take above supplies in a larger quantity than you would expect to use

Nighttime (nocturnal) hypoglycemia

Most parents of little children with diabetes worry about hypoglycemia when they put them to bed for the night. The fears and concerns are justified in that your child is sleeping for a very long period of time and not eating. And you may have had some experience with unpredictable or sudden drops in blood glucose levels. Anyone who has tried to get a sleepy little child to take medicine, eat, or drink during the night knows what a challenge it can be. It is natural to question "Did I give her enough to eat?" "Will the extra activity she had today cause blood glucose to fall?" "Will she show symptoms if there is a problem?" "If I am asleep, will I hear her?" "What happens if I don't?" Sometimes with all your best efforts, low blood glucose does happen at night. However, severe hypoglycemia most often awakens a sleeping child.

Sometimes nocturnal hypoglycemia can be avoided. Severe hypoglycemia can occur when the child falls asleep in the car seat on the way home and is put directly to bed, or when the child falls asleep early, missing bedtime snack.

Children may awaken in the morning with a high or a low blood glucose level. In either case she could be running low during the night. When your child is low, other hormones (epinephrine, cortisol, and glucagon) can automatically kick in and cause high blood glucose later on. Otherwise, the child may just stay low. So doing extra blood checks during the night when you suspect a problem is the best way to solve it.

It is very important for you, as a parent, to get enough sleep so that you can function and be well. Parents who allow themselves to be consistently deprived of sleep have a hard time functioning well. Try to negotiate a schedule with someone to help you do this. Obviously this works best in two-parent families where one partner can take weekends and Wednesday night, and the other partner the other days. Otherwise, sometimes arrangements can be made with willing grandparents, aunts, or uncles to give mom or dad a break once in a while. When the responsibility of nighttime blood checks and treatment falls to one person, he or she can become exhausted.

Ideas for adding protein or fat to bedtime snacks

- Peanut butter
- Lunch meat
- Cottage cheese
- Whole egg
- Cheese stick
- Ice cream
- Yogurt
- Grilled cheese sandwich
- Pizza
- Nuts

Tips for preventing and managing nighttime lows

Make sure that bedtime snack includes not only carbohydrate, but also fat and protein. Fat and protein are slower to be digested, and therefore add some "holding" power for blood glucose levels during the night.

Feeding an infant cake icing on the tip of your finger or pacifier may help keep blood glucose elevated at least for the short term.

Know your child's blood glucose level before bedtime snack. If this number is <100 mg/dl (5.5 mmoles), give the child extra food or milk at the bedtime snack.

Although not always completely reliable, checking your child for sweating and clamminess, twitching, or unusual sounds can give you clues to signs of hypoglycemia.

Purchase a baby monitor to give you peace of mind that you will be able to hear anything unusual. Restless sleep, nightmares, or unusual noises could mean hypoglycemia.

If your child's blood glucose is low and you are unable to get your child to drink the usual juice or soda, you may want to try table syrup, molasses, corn syrup, or jelly.

If blood glucose is low in the morning, it is very likely that it has also been low during the night. (See page 64 and 65, "Nighttime hypoglycemia".)

Check your child's blood glucose before you go to bed on nights when you suspect he could be low. This might be if he had hypoglycemia during the day or before bedtime, if he didn't eat or drink well, if there was unusual activity, or if he has been having a pattern of recurring hypoglycemia.

If your child's blood glucose is low when you are going to bed, provide milk or juice and possibly crackers or another form of carbohydrate and protein. Then check blood glucose again after about fifteen minutes to make sure it has risen. It is a good idea to set the alarm and do a 3 to 4 A.M. blood check after an earlier nighttime low.

When you are anxious about nighttime lows, set the alarm, get up, test and treat your child if necessary, and then go back to bed. This routine, although hard, is better than lying anxious and listening all night.

Plan random nighttime checks once or twice a week at the time when insulin is peaking (working hardest). Try to "catch" a low blood glucose this way. If you are finding the blood glucose is low on random checks, call your diabetes specialist for help.

Consult with your diabetes specialist if your child has frequent or severe hypoglycemia at night.

Try new products that may give a slower release of carbohydrate because they contain cornstarch. Uncooked cornstarch releases glucose into the blood slowly over a period of six or more hours. (See page 45.)

Two such products are called Zbar and Nitebite, and they are offered in different flavors.

Hyperglycemia (high blood glucose)

High blood glucose, like low blood glucose, can occur from an imbalance among insulin, food, and activity. Numbers that are above your target range no doubt will happen, and do not cause an immediate problem. However, problems can occur later from high blood glucose, including poor growth, persistent infections, or other complications of diabetes. This is why it is not a good idea to consistently let a child's blood glucose run very high in order to avoid the lows. It is best to shoot for the target goal of 100–200 mg/dl (5.5-11.1 mmoles) with the understanding that you will get numbers outside of that range. When your child is having high blood glucose, you may notice frequent urination or soaking wet diapers. Your child will also most likely be thirsty and could be irritable.

Tips for managing hyperglycemia in a young child:

Keep up with fluids to prevent dehydration. Give water and sugar-free powdered drink or soda for an older child.

Always feed your child basic meals and snacks, in spite of high numbers. Even though you may be tempted to skip meals or snacks, these nutrients and calories are important for growth. If you do not feed your child, blood glucose levels can fall later on when insulin works hard. On the other hand, if your child doesn't feel like eating all of his food and blood glucose is high it is less likely that he will become hypoglycemic.

Check for ketones if blood glucose is >300 mg/dl (16.6 mmoles). (See Chapter 3.)

Ask your diabetes specialist about correcting a high blood glucose with extra Humalog or Regular insulin at the next dose.

If numbers run consistently out of your goal range for several days, an adjustment in insulin dose, food, or scheduling may be necessary.

High blood glucose and the accompanying large amount of urine can make a difference when your child is toilet training. Young children who have been dry at night can be spared embarrassment if they wear nighttime disposable underwear when blood glucose numbers are running high.

If your child is being a grouch, try to be patient.

Ketoacidosis

When there isn't enough insulin in the body, ketones can form and be present in the blood and urine. The blood can turn acidic, causing nausea, vomiting, dehydration, stomach pains, rapid respiration, fruity smelling breath, coma, and even death if left untreated. This very serious situation, called ketoacidosis, is especially concerning in a very young child. However, it will not come on without warning. You will know from your child's behavior, appearance, and urine and blood test results that he or she is very sick. Call your doctor or diabetes educator immediately when moderate or large ketones are present.

After the initial diagnosis, the most likely time for ketoacidosis to develop is with illness, or if not enough insulin is taken.

Sick days

All parents dread the times when their child is sick. Missed days from work, sleepless nights, and the pain and worry of watching your child not feel well is hard. When your child has diabetes, the anxiety meter increases. In most cases, keeping in mind that some minor adjustments and precautions must be taken, children come through illness without much of a problem. Managing diabetes during sick days adds an additional challenge to the usual cold, flu, ear infection, virus, or other illness. The difficulty is that you usually cannot predict whether glucose levels will go up or down. You will need to be especially watchful during times of illness to prevent or treat high or low blood glucose and ketones.

For most older children and adults who are ill, glucose levels rise due to the release of stress hormones and the release of glycogen, which is a form of stored glucose. Infants and young children do not have the ability to store much glycogen in their body, and therefore don't have it to release if they need it. Therefore, blood glucose levels in young children may run low instead of high as you might expect in an older child or adult during an illness or fever.

Illness itself will affect the blood glucose. If there is nausea, vomiting, or diarrhea, blood glucose levels may be low due to poor absorption of food or not enough food being taken in. On the other hand, fever and infection, such as an ear infection, can cause numbers to skyrocket. There is no way to predict which way things will go. There is often concern that the medication (such as antibiotics or cold medicine) will cause blood glucose levels to run high. However, usually it is the illness itself that causes the release of stress hormones that cause the highs. Diabetes can be unpredictable in this way, so you need to learn to just go with the flow. If blood glucose levels run low, offer carbohydrates and reduce insulin doses. If blood glucose levels are high, you will need to increase insulin doses. In any case you will need to monitor urine ketones, watch for signs of dehydration, and keep in close contact with your diabetes specialist.

In the past, the traditional BRAT (bananas, rice, applesauce, toast) diet has been recommended for diarrhea by most pediatric care providers. However, the new guidelines by the American Academy of Pediatrics note that it is low in energy density, protein, and fat and is not the diet of choice for children with diarrhea. This is also true for children who are vomiting. Better foods are complex carbohydrates such as rice and cereals, lean meats, yogurt, fruit, and vegetables.

Signs of dehydration
- thirst
- sunken eyes
- dry cracked lips
- dry mouth
- skin that remains pinched up after it's pinched
- concentrated urine

Diarrhea treatment
Give specially formulated products with electrolytes for children, found in your pharmacy. (For example, Kao lectrolyte, a flavored powder is mixed with water to replace fluids and minerals lost in diarrhea and vomiting.)

Give fluids that contain carbohydrate and sodium, such as Sprite, 7-Up, broth, or soup.

Offer hard candy, Popsicles, glucose tablets, and complex carbohydrates for hypoglycemia.

Tips for managing sick days

The most important thing to do when your child is ill is to check the urine for ketones. If ketones are present, call your diabetes specialist. The sooner you treat the ketones, the better your child will feel.

Urine ketones should be checked as often as every two to four hours, or whenever the child urinates, until ketones are negative.

Frequent blood glucose monitoring is necessary during illness (at least every two to four hours) to carefully monitor and treat upward or downward trends.

During illness, the usual insulin dose may need to be adjusted.

Always give your child his insulin. It is important to check with your diabetes specialist about the dose, but even if he is vomiting, he will need insulin.

Do not wait for patterns of highs or lows to make insulin adjustments during illness.

If your child vomits more than once, notify your diabetes specialist. Repeated vomiting in a young child may require intravenous (IV) fluids at a hospital to recover.

It can be tricky to get your hypoglycemic infant to eat or drink when he is sick. You can try cake icing or syrup on your finger or a nipple, or table sugar on the tip of your finger. Older children may do well with glucose tablets, Popsicles, sherbet, or candy.

Encourage fluids, specifically one ounce or more every twenty minutes. If your child is not eating, alternate sugar-free with sweetened choices.

CHAPTER 5

Special Issues of Infants and Toddlers

ALTHOUGH ALL STAGES of a child's development have their charms, for many people infancy and toddlerhood are the favorites. Only a baby can turn a group of mature, serious adults into silly, cooing, playful clowns.

There is no other time of life where development proceeds as quickly and with as much intensity as during infancy. During infancy, babies explore everything through touch, smell, taste, sight, and hearing, and progress from:

- sleeping only a few hours at a time to sleeping through the night;
- breast- or bottle-feeding to drinking from a cup;
- learning to eat solid food from a spoon to picking up finger foods to feed themselves;
- babbling to forming words, then putting words together;
- becoming social and smiling to initiating contact with a playmate;
- total reliance on others for care to making needs and wants known to others.

This is also a period of time when children are building a sense of trust in their world and in those around them. This trusting relationship comes from having their needs met by those who take care of them. They learn to communicate that they are hungry, cold, wet, etc., and they trust that when they do, their needs will be met.

Impact of diabetes
Your baby with diabetes should grow and develop normally. In spite of this, some of the developmental steps of normal infancy are

naturally impacted by diabetes management. Diabetes management issues play into normal development, and normal developmental issues affect diabetes care.

Your baby may need to eat or drink when she is not hungry or thirsty. It can be tricky trying to get your young child to eat or drink, yet you know this is important in preventing hypoglycemia. (See "How Little Ones Eat," on page 27.) Your baby may also need treatment for hypoglycemia, and you may have difficulty getting food or drink into her.

Your baby will have to have frequent injections, finger pricks, and blood work at doctor appointments. All of these will eventually become a way of life and are accepted to some degree by most children. However, it is not normal for a child to have to have these intrusive sticks done, and if not well handled, can cause your child to be less trusting of the world. If she grows to believe that someone can come out of anywhere to stick or pinch her, sleeping or otherwise, she may be less likely to sleep well. This is why it is usually recommended that anything uncomfortable or intrusive be done in a special area of the house (but not her bed). (See "Helpful Hints at Injection Times," on page 33.)

When your baby first develops diabetes, she will have reached a certain level of development. It is quite common, however, for children to regress in some of their developmental steps for a while after the diagnosis. For example, a child who has quit sucking her thumb or using a security object may once again need to do so. Or if a child is making progress in potty training she may backslide to having accidents partially due to having high blood glucose. Or another child who has begun to take first walking steps may put those first steps on hold for a while. This is common, as your young child only has so much energy and needs it directed into recovering physically and emotionally from the effect of diabetes and hospitalization. It is usually easily overcome in time.

As long as your child has enough insulin to meet the needs of all cells in the body, growth should be normal. However, if your child does not get enough insulin over long periods of time, the rate of her growth may drop.

Toddlers usually eat three meals and three snacks a day, but may require extra snacks to balance extra activity. Guidelines are available from your diabetes educator.

One of the usual goals of parents of infants is to stretch the nighttime feeding intervals as long as possible until baby eventually sleeps through the night. However, when baby has diabetes, due to the need for more frequent feedings and limited capacity to take in large quantities of food, your baby will probably continue to need a nighttime feeding, at least until she is able to take in cereal along with her milk at bedtime. Usually cereal is added at around five months, and higher protein foods such as cottage cheese, egg yolk, or yogurt can be added at around seven months.

If baby is breast-feeding, breast milk may be pumped and frozen or stored for supplementation and later use. Try not to wean baby from breast-feeding at or around the time of diagnosis. There is plenty of time to wean after life settles down.

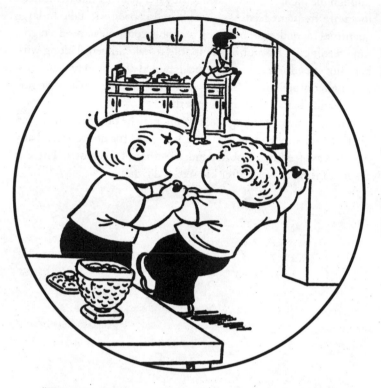

"Wait! Dummy! Put the candy in your mouth FIRST! THEN ask if you can have a piece!"

CHAPTER 6

Special Issues of Preschoolers

THE TYPICAL PRESCHOOLER is delightful, energetic, and demanding. He may push every limit and try every ounce of your patience. It is this age that can test your endurance, as your child explores every corner of his environment.

The preschool-age child is just busy. He is into everything, wants everything, and is sporadic in his growth, activity, and eating. Developmentally, his strength increases and fine motor coordination improves, and he is able to brush his own teeth with help, draw, color, cut, count, balance on one foot, jump, and define words. Word games, books, and stories become fun as he has a fascination with words. (Dr. Seuss lives!) However, attention span is usually short, and he is easily distracted.

In spite of the short attention span, the preschooler can sit still longer to eat or play. He enjoys fun foods, finger foods, special foods. Falling asleep is easy and he can console himself with a security object such as a blanket. Usually he will sleep through the night, and may nap one to two times a day. Toilet training comes when he is ready.

At age three or more, he becomes social, and looks for the approval and affection of his parent or caretaker. On the other hand, he is also frequently negative. He has a great desire to have his body intact and the wholeness of his body is important to him. Therefore, the use of bandages is quite important. (See page 34.)

Children around the age of four are good at "magical thinking." Things happen without relationships. Inanimate objects can take on lives and personalities of their own. For example, you may hear Trisha say "The stick hit me!" She also absorbs the attitudes and feelings shown by others toward her, and will select behaviors that fit into these expectations. Behavior is molded by the expectations of parents and caregivers.

Impact of diabetes

In addition to benefiting from many of the tips listed in "Special Issues of Infants and Toddlers" (Chapter 5), preschoolers with diabetes have some unique qualities.

Although preschool children have reasonably good verbal skills, they do not understand why they must have injections, finger sticks, and food restrictions. They may see these procedures as punishments. Therefore, it is important to stress that all of these "musts" are because "I love you" and "to keep you healthy!" Your child may still not really understand this but it is more positive than the message "because you are sick."

Treat hypoglycemia with whatever you think your preschooler will easily take. One mother, who knows her child likes juice boxes, keeps them around exclusively for treating low blood glucose. Keep on hand a ready supply of those foods and beverages that you know your child will be most likely to take.

Preschoolers are very afraid of intrusive procedures. Loss of control can be frightening for a child. Helping them to hold still by hugging is a good idea for injections or blood draws. Then let them know that they were brave and/or did a great job of holding still (see Chapter 3).

Allow your child to participate in the process of monitoring and injections. the child can help to select the space, cleanse the skin, push the button, etc. Make the procedure as quick, efficient, and matter-of-fact as possible. He may need a reasonable time to prepare himself, but the less time to argue, negotiate, barter, or bribe, the better!

Try to maintain a cheerful, fun-loving, well-organized daily routine! (This tip was actually offered by one parent, although feedback from other parents suggests "You've got to be kidding!")

It is important to try to match insulin type, peak, and action as closely as possible to the way the child naturally eats. For example, Johnny might not eat breakfast well at all, but will then eat a terrific lunch. Using much of a fast-acting insulin like Humalog or

Regular in the morning would not match his eating habits. (See Chapter 3.)

If your child is not eating well, offer milk, juice, or other beverages that contain carbohydrates. Sometimes, if you offer the food twenty to thirty minutes later, your child may actually eat. (See Chapter 3 for help with finicky eaters.)

Encourage your child to "play out" his feelings and concerns about diabetes. This is how children deal with their worries. Puppets or figures that represent your family may be useful for Johnny to play out feelings about injections, finger pricks, or a hospitalization. As a parent, participating in the play, or at least listening carefully to it, may tell you a lot about what your child is thinking and feeling.

CHAPTER 7

Day Care and Preschool Issues

ONE OF THE hardest things for a parent to do under normal circumstances is to entrust a young child's care to someone else. Most parents are comfortable with a baby-sitter in the home for short periods of time, but to take a young child out of the home on a regular basis to accommodate a work schedule, or for other reasons, can be worrisome. When the young child has diabetes, the worry can be compounded. The biggest issue is in educating caregivers about the signs and treatment for hypoglycemia, the monitoring of blood glucose levels, and establishing guidelines about when to call for help.

Centers that are federally funded are obligated to provide services to everyone, regardless of any physical, developmental, emotional, or other health impairments. However, there are few federally funded programs for infants, toddlers, and preschool-age children. Most day care centers and preschools are privately owned, and in the past have fallen under the legal umbrella of private business, and therefore could be selective about who they could take into their programs. Although most centers are willing to take a child with medical conditions into their program, there are both insurance and safety factors to be considered. These concerns may make child care facilities reluctant to take children with certain medical conditions. There has recently been some challenging of these concerns through the courts for specific preschools.

The Americans with Disabilities Act is civil rights legislation designed to protect people with mental or physical disabilities from discrimination based upon disability. Title 21 prohibits discrimination on the basis of disability by public accommodations and requires places of public accommodation and commercial facilities to be designed, constructed, and altered in compliance with certain guidelines. Public accommodations include a variety of businesses, such as restaurants, hotels, retail establishments, hospitals, and child care centers.

The Americans with Disabilities Act states that public accommodations, including child care centers, must make reasonable modifications in policies, practices, and procedures in order to accommodate those with disabilities. A modification is not required if it would "fundamentally alter" the goods or services of the institution or place "undue burden" (significant difficulty or expense).

Possible changes that child care centers must provide may include

- Revision of policies and procedures
- Curriculum adaptations
- Removal of physical barriers
- Provision of additional staff training
- Alteration of staffing patterns
- Provision of certain adaptive equipment

Things you should expect from your child care provider

OPEN COMMUNICATION. You and your provider should seek open communication, including frequent and full updates on your child's progress and problems. Explain clearly and carefully your wishes and expectations about how your child will be cared for. Your provider should welcome your questions and ask questions about how he or she can help your child.

OPEN ACCESS. As a parent, you must be welcome to drop in any time, even without calling. Providers should allow parents to make phone calls to check in during the day. You should both work out the best times for these calls and decide how many are reasonable.

SAFETY. Providers should take all possible precautions to keep children safe.

HONESTY, TRUST, AND CONFIDENCE. Commitments made by both parent and provider should be kept.

ACCEPTANCE OF PARENTS' WISHES. Providers should abide by parents' wishes on matters of safety, discipline, food, toilet training, adult smoking, and dealing with behavior problems.

ADVANCE NOTICE OF ANY CHANGES IN CARE. For both parent and provider, when changes in care or routine are anticipated, it is best to communicate this immediately.

ASSURANCE THAT EVERYONE IN CONTACT WITH THE CHILD IS TRUSTWORTHY, PROPERLY TRAINED, AND SUPERVISED. Most programs have staff who are inexperienced in caring for children with diabetes. Therefore, much time is required to educate staff so that everyone is comfortable with the issues in such a situation. The primary issue for a child in day care is that the staff be able to recognize the signs and know how to treat hypoglycemia in a consistent way. Begin with a conference involving parents and all staff involved in the child's care. Develop a written plan of care with input from both parents and staff alike, including both the regular day's routine and the diabetes routine. As you develop your plan, you may want to consider the following inclusions:

A WRITTEN PLAN OF CARE: Your plan should include the following information:

1. Educate the school personnel who will have contact with your child.

Signs of hypoglycemia (child's usual signs_____)
- crying
- irritable
- sweaty, clammy
- shaking
- hungry
- sleepy
- uncoordinated
- restless
- twitching
- unresponsive

Reasons for hypoglycemia
- not enough food
- delayed meal or snack
- too much insulin
- extra activity

Preferred and emergency treatment for hypoglycemia
- where supplies for hypoglycemia are located_____

_____

• how much and what foods and beverages to provide

FOOD   AMOUNT

_____   _____
_____   _____
_____   _____
_____   _____
_____   _____

• test blood glucose
• glucagon— to be used when child is unable to eat, drink, or
  swallow: Dose is 0.5 mg for children under six years
• designated person to give glucagon _____

General information about diabetes and its treatment
• causes of diabetes
• signs of high blood glucose: increased thirst, frequent urination, dehydration
• urine testing; meaning of ketones
• balancing insulin, food, and activity
• normal activity/nap plan
• communicating changes in activity

Blood glucose monitoring
• when to test blood glucose
   regular times _____
   special times _____
   signs of hypoglycemia _____
• how to test blood glucose
• action values
• when to act to treat low blood glucose _____
   action _____
   when to call about high blood glucose _____
• record keeping
• communication with others and parents of values

Food issues
• general meal plan information
• meal and snack times _____
• food plan/snack foods _____
• special occasion foods _____

2. Establishing a plan of communication

when to contact parent _____

where to call _____

emergency phone numbers _____

Helpful Resources

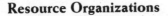

Resource Organizations

American Association of Diabetes Educators (AADE)
100 West Monroe
4th Floor
Chicago, IL 60603

312/424-2426

Website: http://www.aadenet.org

Call for information regarding pediatric diabetes education support in your area.

American Diabetes Association (ADA)
ADA National Service Center
1660 Duke St.
Alexandria, VA 22314

1-800/232-2472

703/549-1500

Website: http://www.diabetes.org

Call for membership information, for state and local affiliate activities and programs, publications, and for programs recognized as having met standards for diabetes care and education in your area.

The American Dietetic Association
216 W. Jackson Blvd.
Suite 3800
Chicago, IL 60606-6995

1-800/877-1600
312/899-0040

Website: http:www.eatright.org

Call for information regarding pediatric nutrition and diabetes management support services in your area.

The Juvenile Diabetes Foundation International (JDF)
120 Wall St.
New York, NY 10005

1-800/223-1138

Website: http://www.jdfcure.com

Call for membership information, publications, and local chapter activities and programs.

National Association for the Education of Young Children (NAEYC)
1509 16th St. NW
Washington, DC 20036

1-800/424-2460
202/232-8777

Website: http://www.naeyc.org

Other Websites:

National Institute of Diabetes and Digestive and Kidney Diseases (NIDDK)
http://niddk.nih.gov
This site offers access to the government's diabetes database, along with a diabetes dictionary and other basic research information.

Children with Diabetes
http://www.childrenwithdiabetes.com
The online community for kids, families, and adults with Type 1

diabetes. User-friendly information featuring chat rooms for children and parents, a message board, up-to-date news clips and links to Usenet newsgroups.

Online Resources for Diabetics
http://www.cruzio.com/~mendosa/faq.html
This page provides access to hundreds of diabetes related sites.

Helpful Publications
For Parents:
Growing Up with Diabetes, by Alicia McAuliffe. Chronimed Publishing, 1998.

Raising a Child with Diabetes, by Linda Siminerio and Jean Betschart. American Diabetes Association, 1995.

Sweet Kids: How to Balance Diabetes Control & Good Nutrition with Family Peace, by Betty Brackenridge & Richard Rubin. American Diabetes Association, 1996.

The Ten Keys to Helping Your Child Grow Up with Diabetes, by Tim Wysocki. American Diabetes Association, 1997.

For Young Children:
Sarah and Puffle, by Linnea Mulder. Magination Press, 1992.

A Magic Ride in Foozbah Land, book and audiotape, by Jean Betschart. Chronimed Publishing, 1995.

D Is for Dudley Dragon and Diabetes. by Janice Zack. 1992. For information, call (540) 224-4620.

Index